My First Colonoscopy

By Bob Joseph & Mal Karlin

This book my be purchased in bulk for promotional, educational, or business use. Please contact Mal Karlin at 212-779-3375, malkarlin@gmail.com or Bob Joseph at 917-881-4345, Bob@andbob.com

ISBN- 978-0-692-17566-8
978-0-692-16854-7

Published by IngramSpark
For The Him and Me Project

DEDICATED TO OUR WIVES DIANA AND VALERIE WHO CONTINUE TO PUT UP WITH US ASSHOLES.
YOU'RE SQUEEZING ME.
HIM & ME

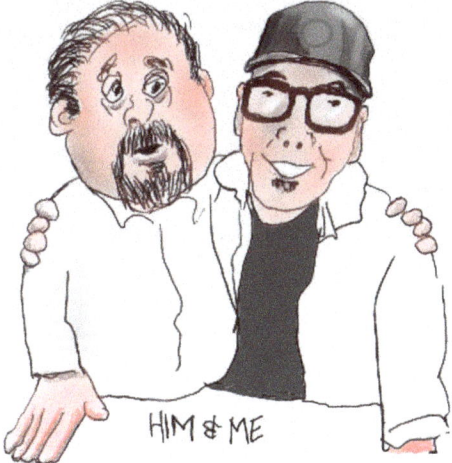

Couples Colonoscopy
I CALL THIS ILLUSION
"IN ONE END AND OUT THE OTHER"
NEXT STOP . . . VEGAS !!

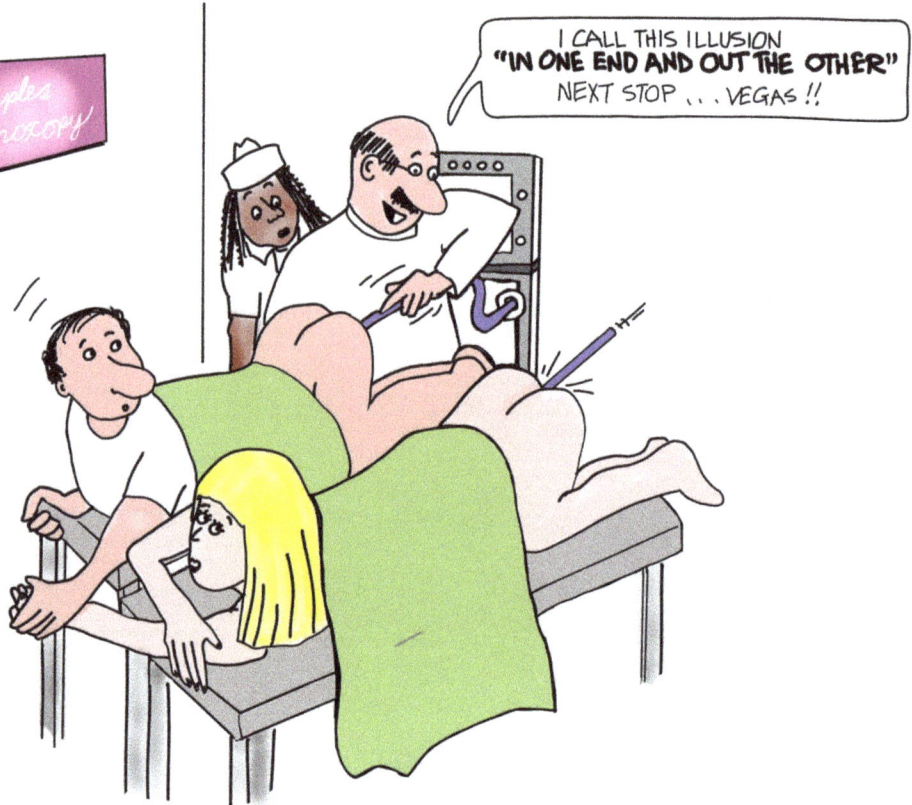

What you can look forward to in the near future
from Bob Joseph and Mal Karlin:

My First Grey Hair
My First Double Chin
My Wife's First Hot Flash
My First Divorce
My First Balloon Angioplasty
My First Cataract
My First Bout with the Gout
My First Knee Replacement
My First Hip Replacement
My First "Where Did You Put My______?"
My First Grandchild (can do no wrong!)
My First Day of Retirement
My First Day Back to Work (at a fraction of the pay)
My Second Wife's First Facelift
MY FIRST HEARING AID!

HOW 'BOUT A COURTESY FLUSH.

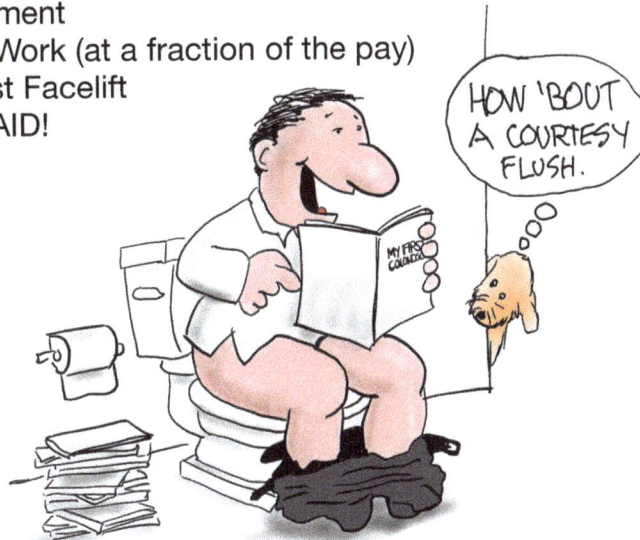

My First Colonoscopy

SAY HELLO TO MY NEW STUDENT NURSE, STACY... SHE WILL BE OBSERVING TODAY'S PROCEDURE.

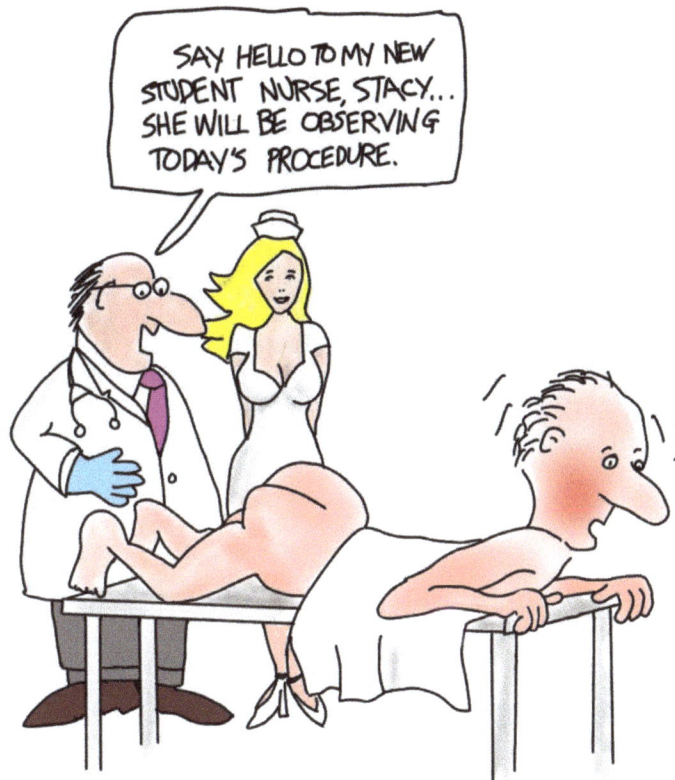

I've had many fearful firsts
In my life so far,
Like my first day of school
When I hid in the car.

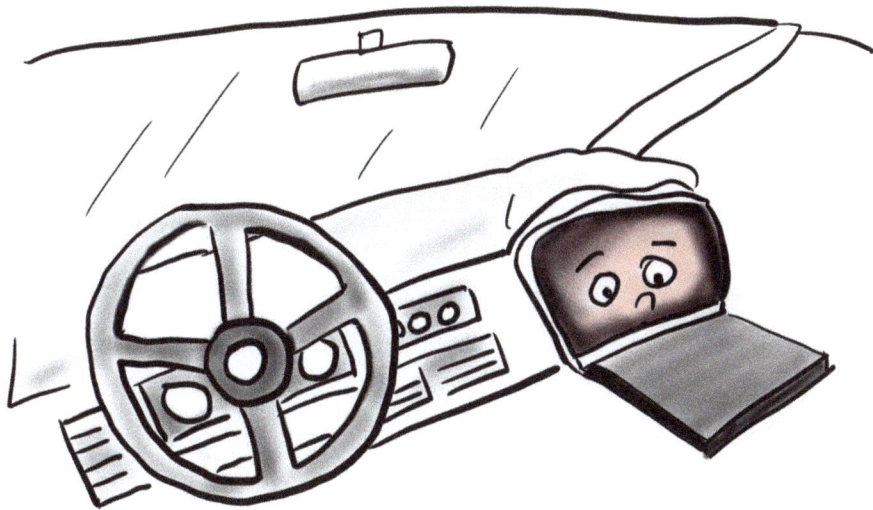

And the first time at the dentist,
I shut my mouth for an hour!
But what could I do,
I was a kid with no power.

VERY FUNNY BOBBY, NOT THE CRAZY GLUE AGAIN?

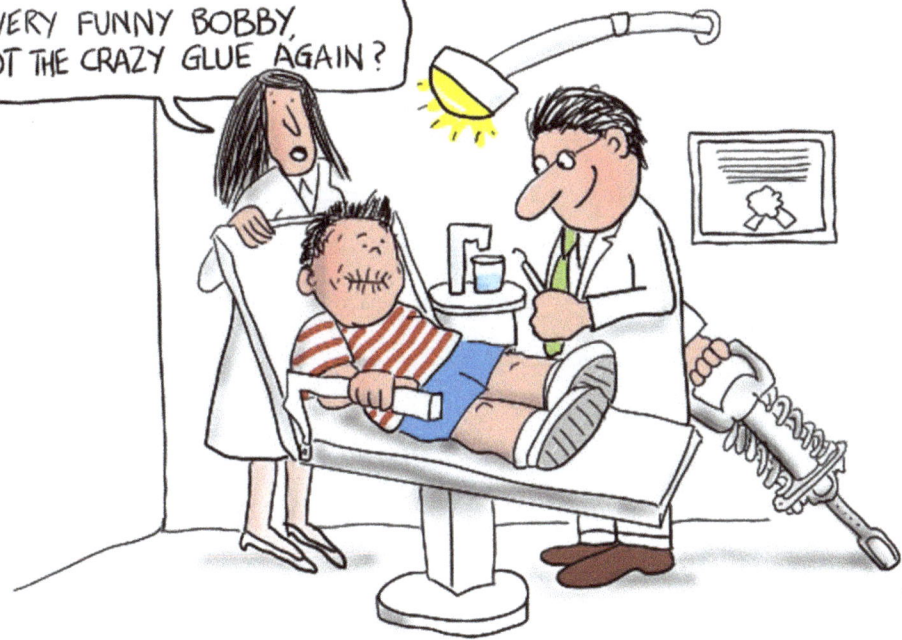

But when I turned 45
I had a new first that I feared,
A long rubber hose
That would get shoved up my rear.

HE'S HERE TO CATCH YOUR TEETH IN CASE I PROBE TOO FAR.

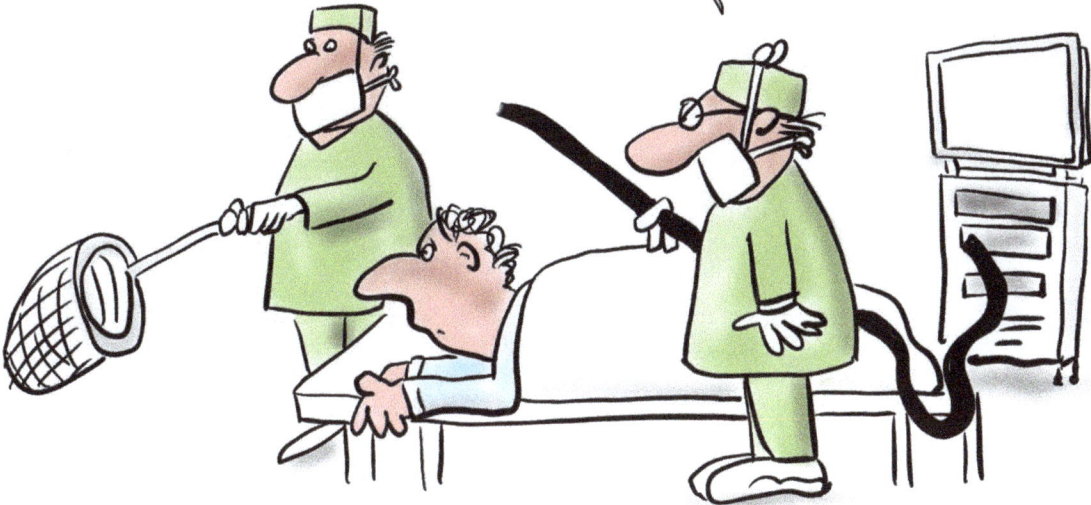

I had plenty of fears,
Like would my sphincter behave?
Would they find scary monsters
In those mazes and caves?

CHAMBER
OF
HORRORS

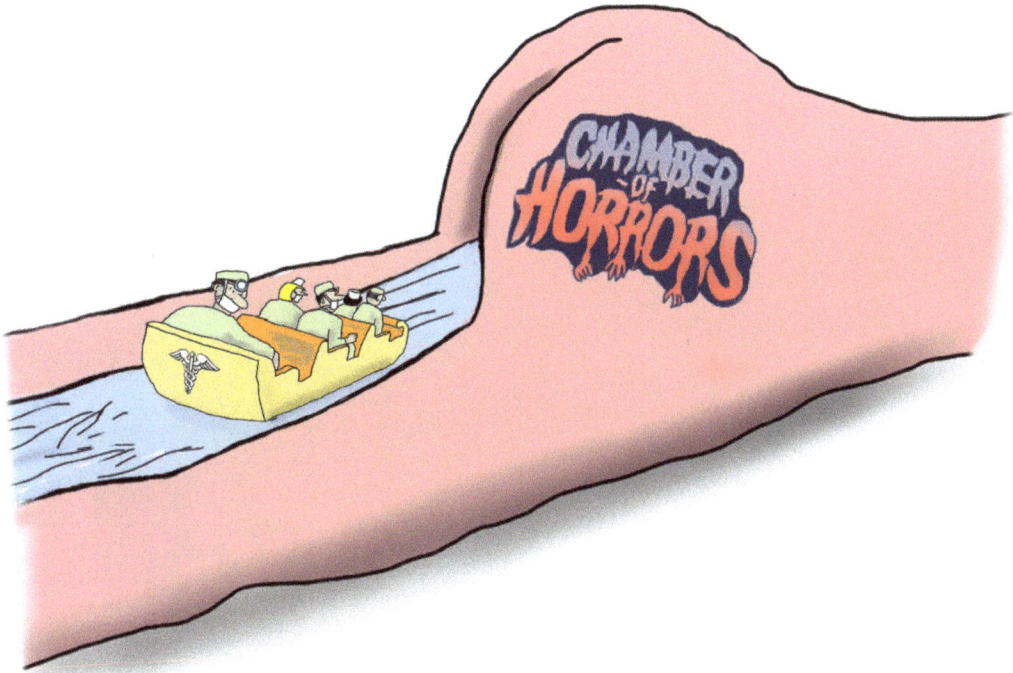

Co-lon-os-co-py has many syllables,
"Ass" you can see,
The first time I heard it
Was a spelling bee on TV.

CAN YOU SAY IT IN A SENTENCE?
SPELLING BEE

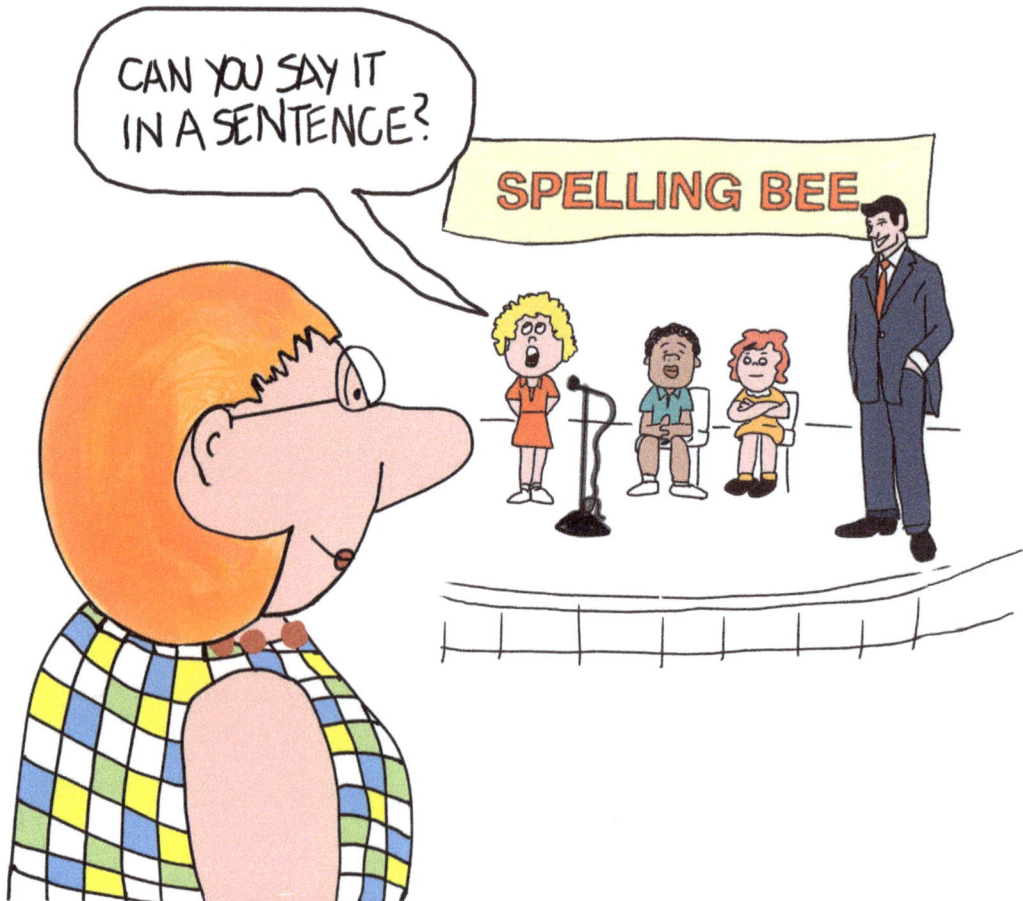

They had to say it and spell it
And say it again –
Meanwhile I'm gonna get
Poked like a pig in a pen!

I'D LIKE TO GIVE MR. HARDWOOD A COLONOSCOPY.
SPELLING BEE

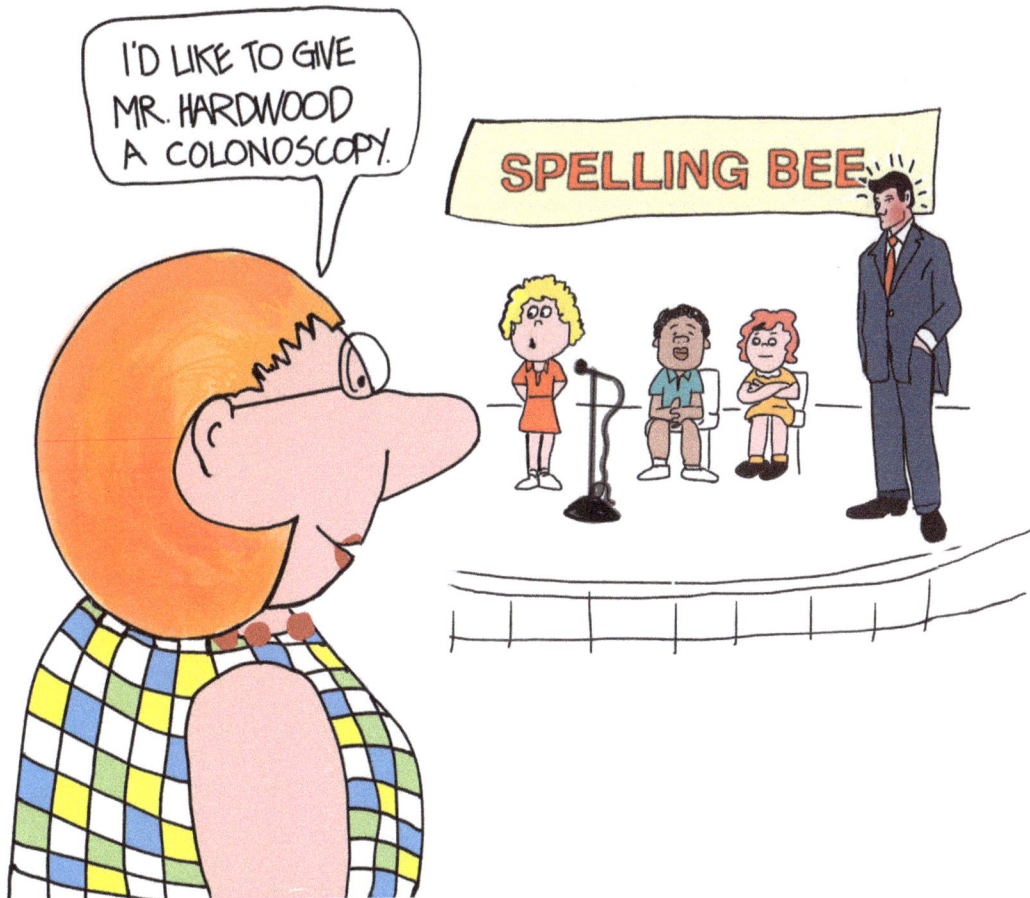

My rectum was so scared
I thought my anus would shut!
The thought of a colonoscopy
Sent shivers up my you-know-what!

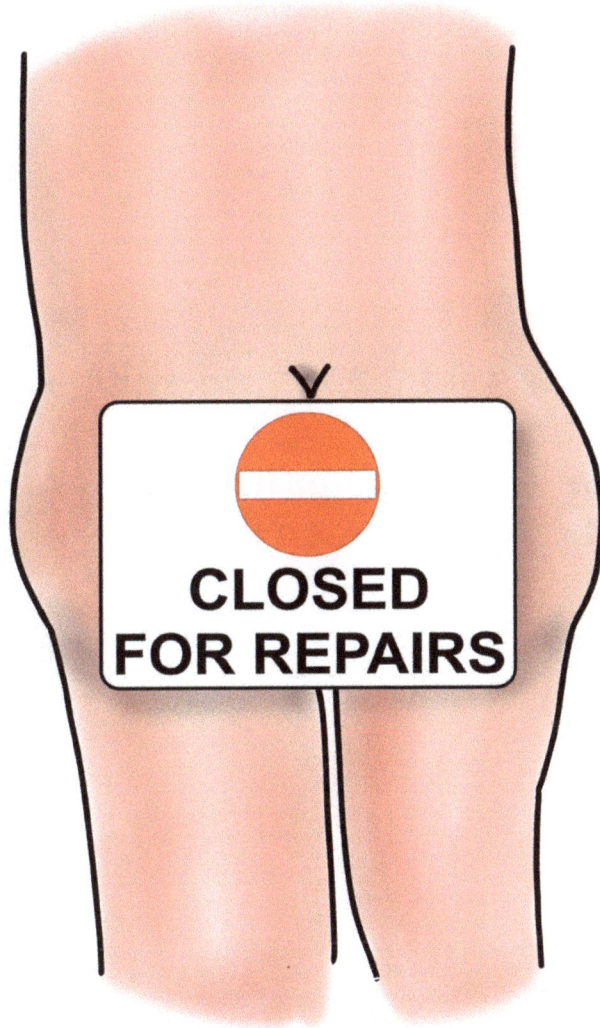

CLOSED
FOR REPAIRS

Friends said, "Don't worry,"
My son said, "Do it, Dad!"
My wife who never had one
Said, "It can't be so bad!"

A COLONOSCO-PEE ??
SURE BITCH, I CAN DO THAT!!

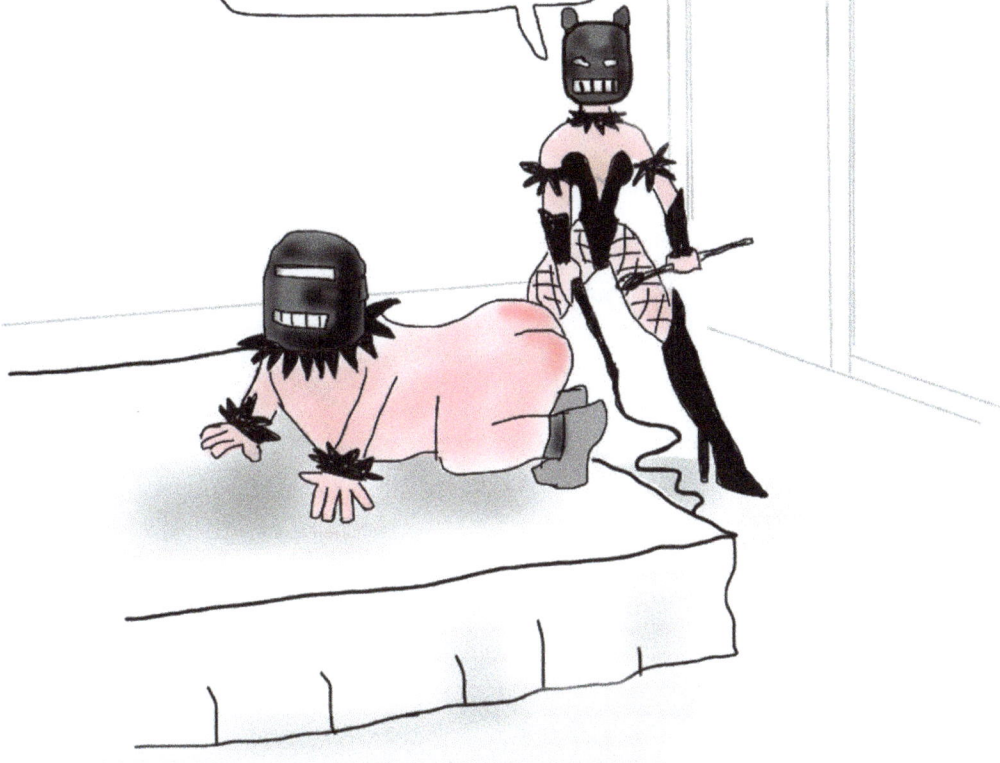

The prep, I was told
Was the most difficult part.
Warned, be near a toilet
Before the *'Fizzzzusgenning'* starts!

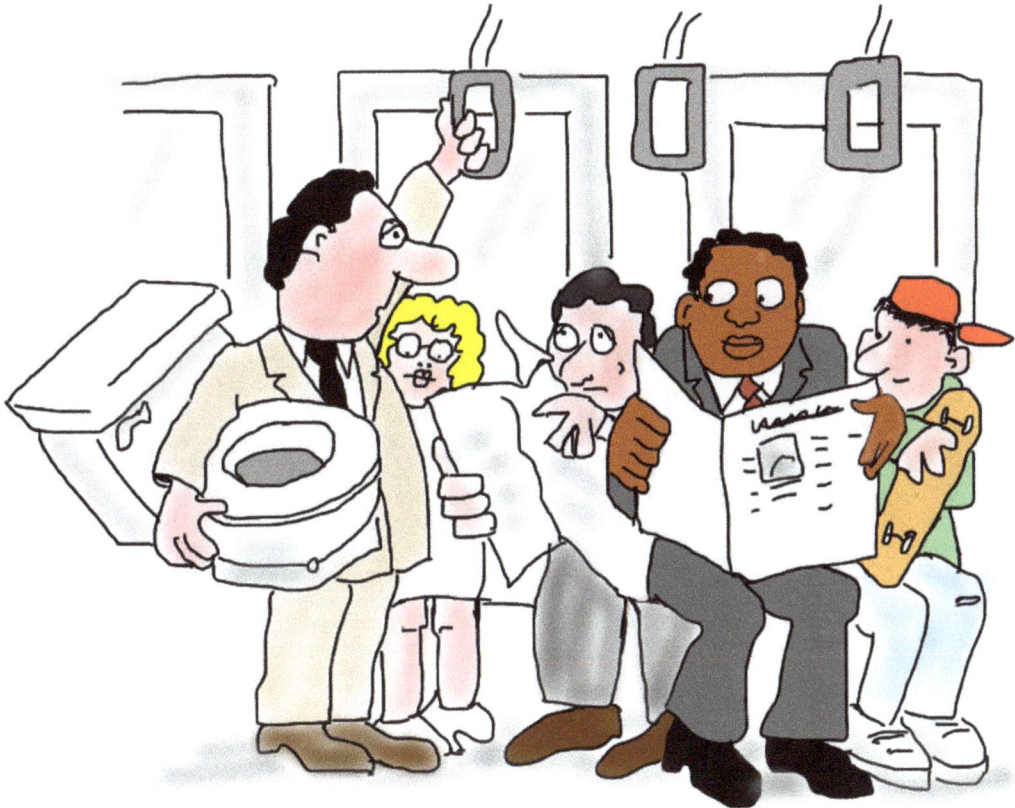

That will be followed by a chorus
Of rat-a-tat-tats,
So run like a sprinter
If you don't want to splat.
*(HINT: Hold the cuffs of your pant legs,
to avoid that).*

GIMEE ALL YOUR SHIT!! AND DON'T FORGET WHAT'S HIDING IN YOUR CUFF.
I SMELL SOMETHING

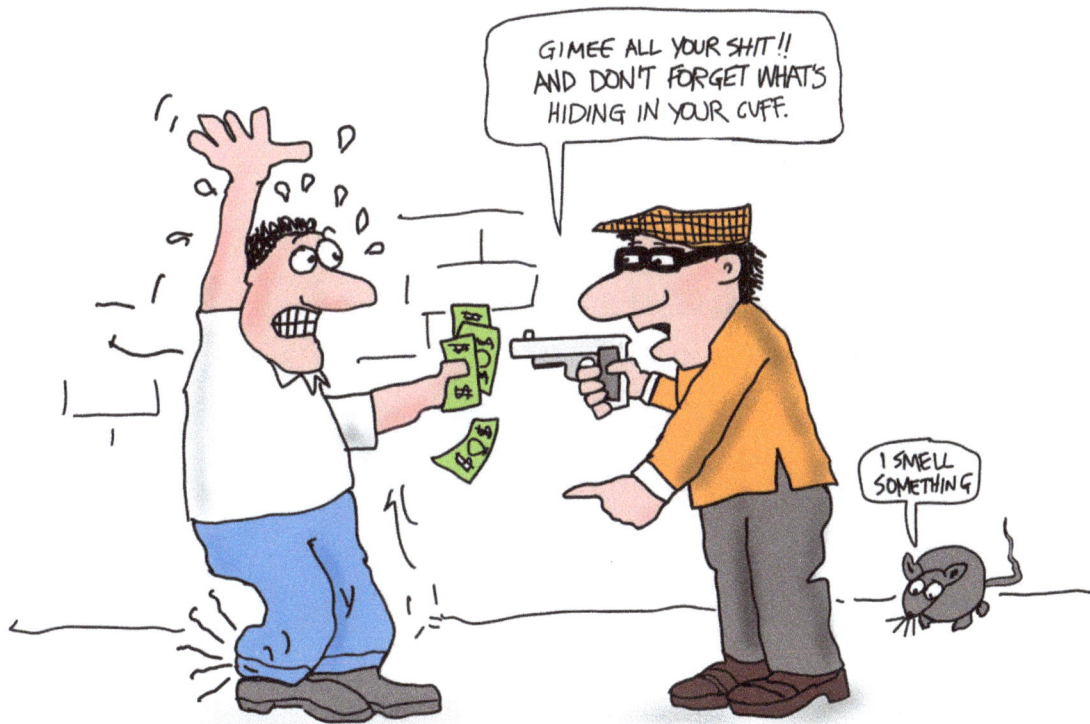

The instructions said
I could eat Jello,
But LARGE TYPE warned
Don't be a dumb fellow.

TOILET PAPER OR PLASTIC?
SUPERMARKET
WEEKLY SPECIALS
JELLO

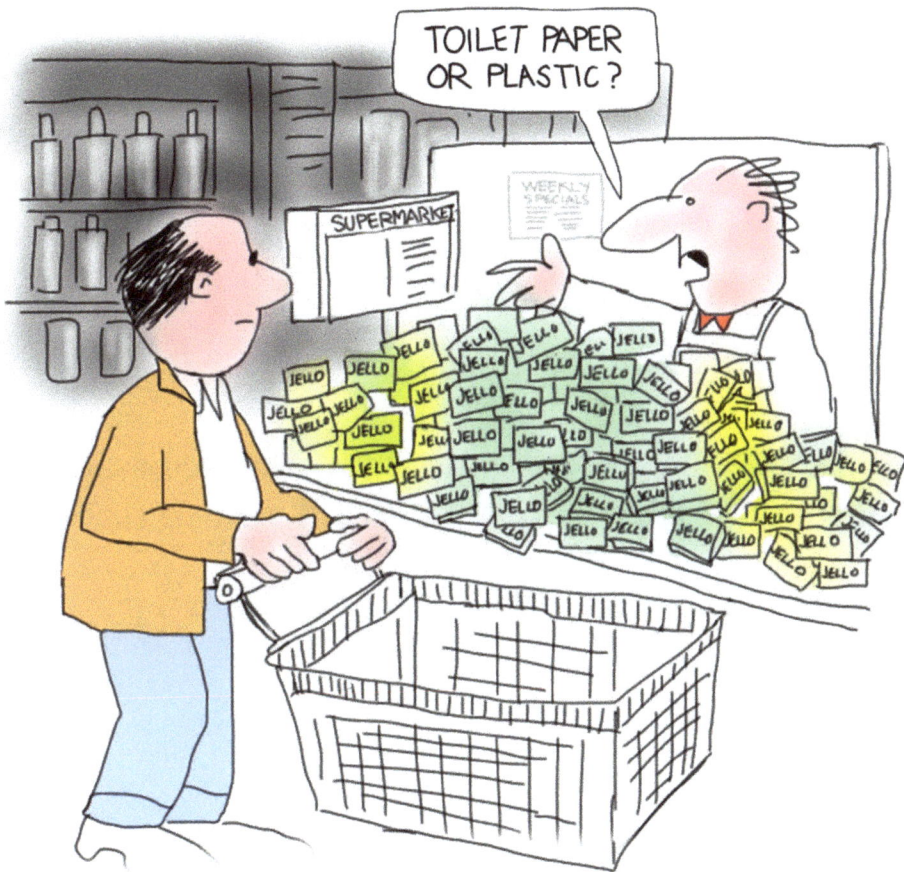

Don't eat any Jello
That's purple or red,
Or they'll think it's blood in your stool
And give you a week till you're dead.

WHAT PART OF **NOTHING RED** DIDN'T YOU UNDERSTAND?
PROCEDURE ROOM

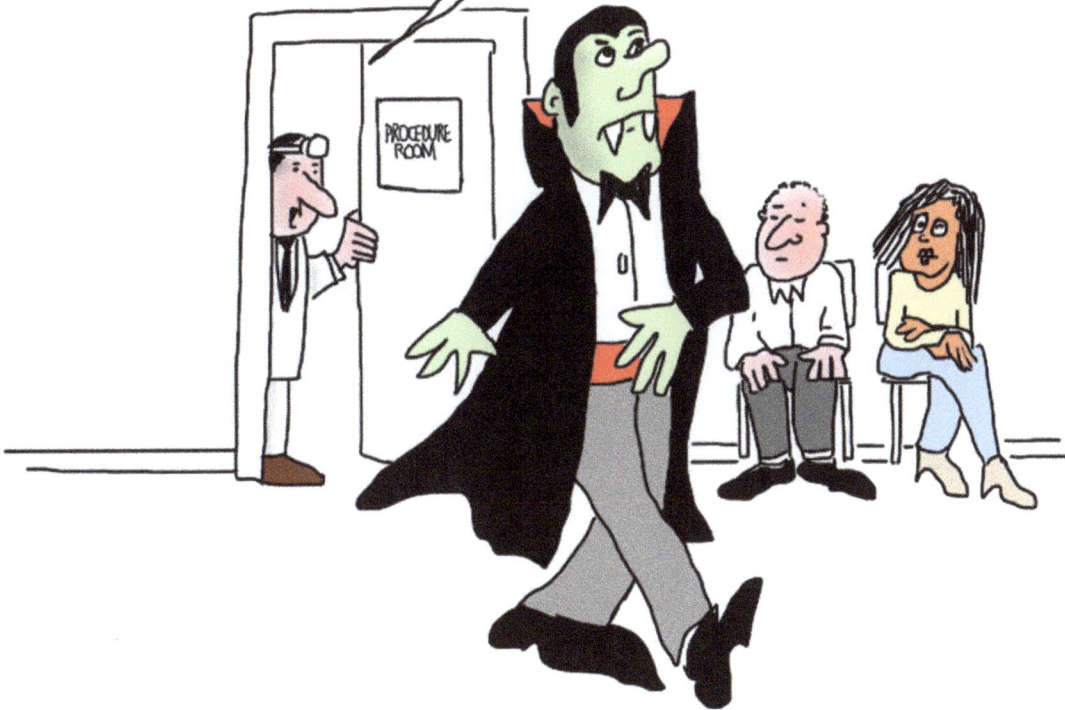

I was more than embarrassed,
Scared shitless and crazed!
Couldn't we postpone it,
'Till past the holidays?

NURSE, TELL RECEPTION I'M RUNNING A LITTLE BEHIND!

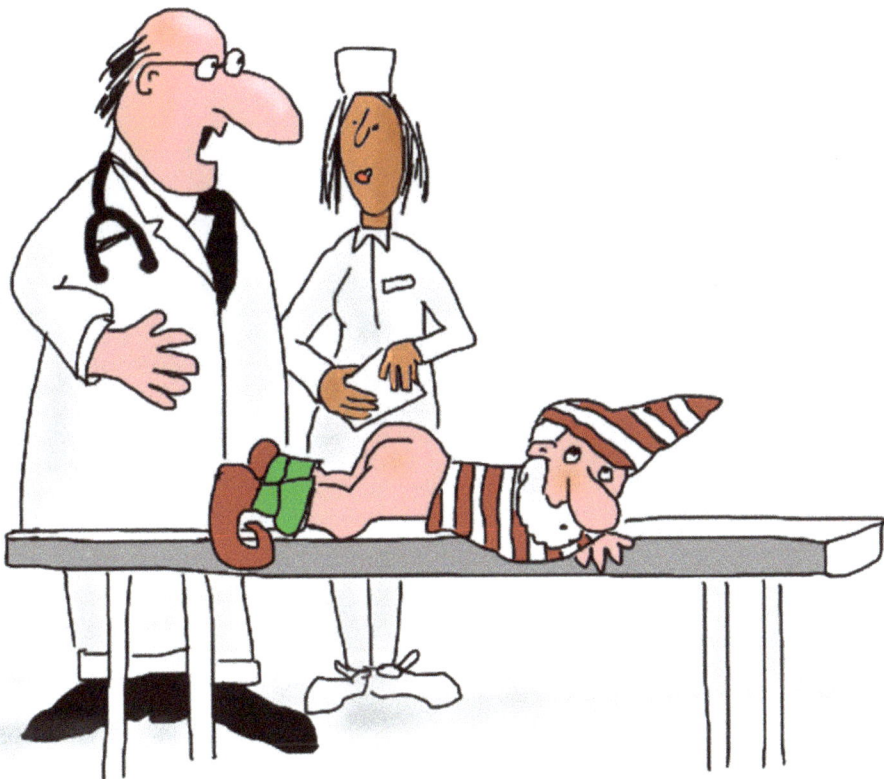

It was "colonoscopy time!"
And it was getting real scary.
Would they shave my behind
'Cause it was kind of hairy?

AND IF I SHAVE YOUR BALLS IT'S COVERED BY INSURANCE!
SHAVE FOAM

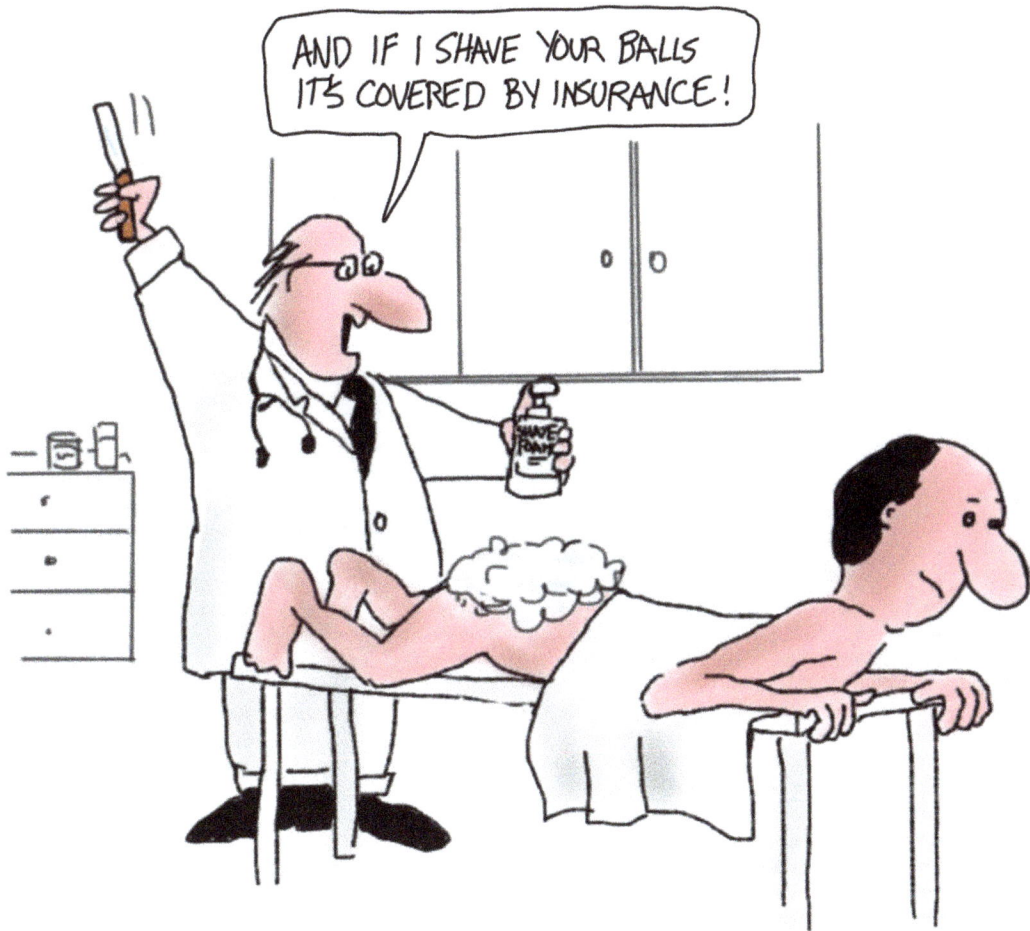

The doc said, "Trust me Bob,
You won't even feel sore,
Lots of brave guys
Have done this before."

SINCE BEING LISTED AS A TOP GASTRO HE'S BEEN A ROYAL PAIN IN THE ASS.
RECEPTION

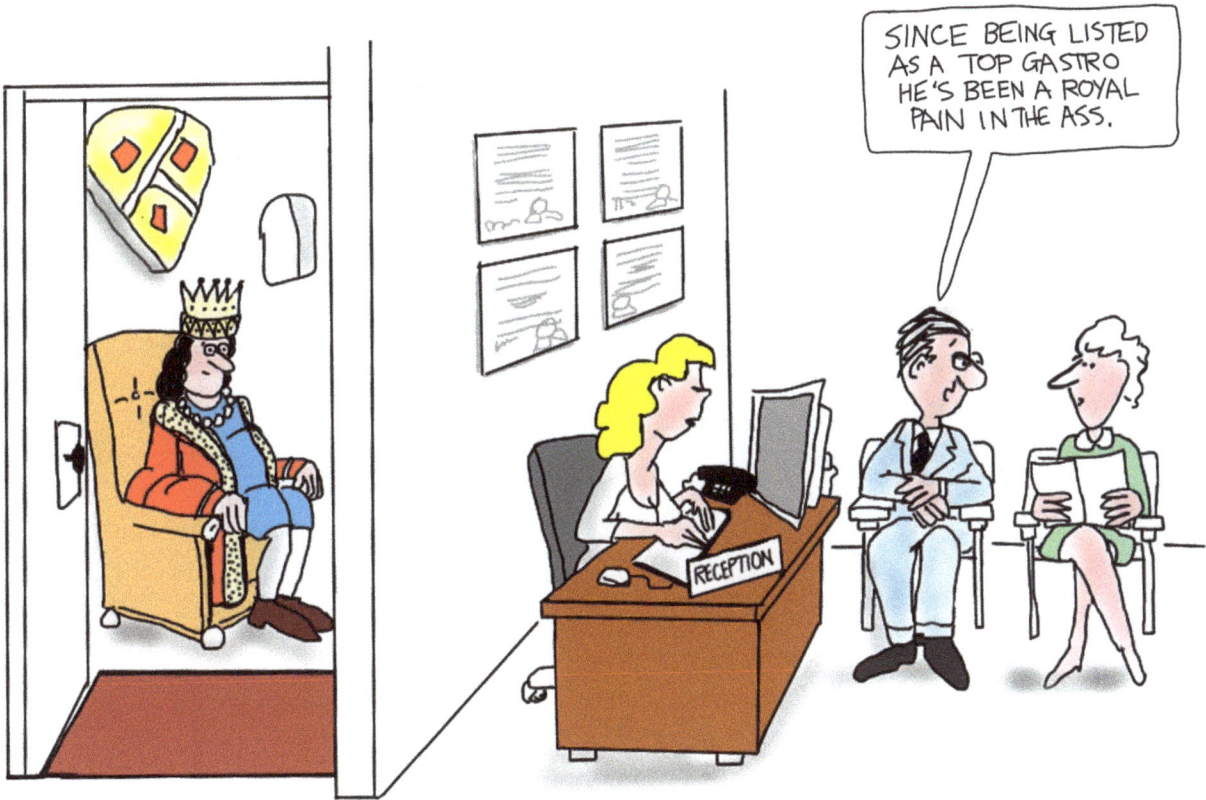

Was Colin Powell brave
When he had his done?
Being named after your colon
Couldn't have been fun!

GENTLEMEN, WE HAVE LOCATED THE WEAPONS OF MASS DESTRUCTION!
FART
FART
FART
FART
S.B.D.'s
IT'S THOSE DAMN CHICK PEAS!

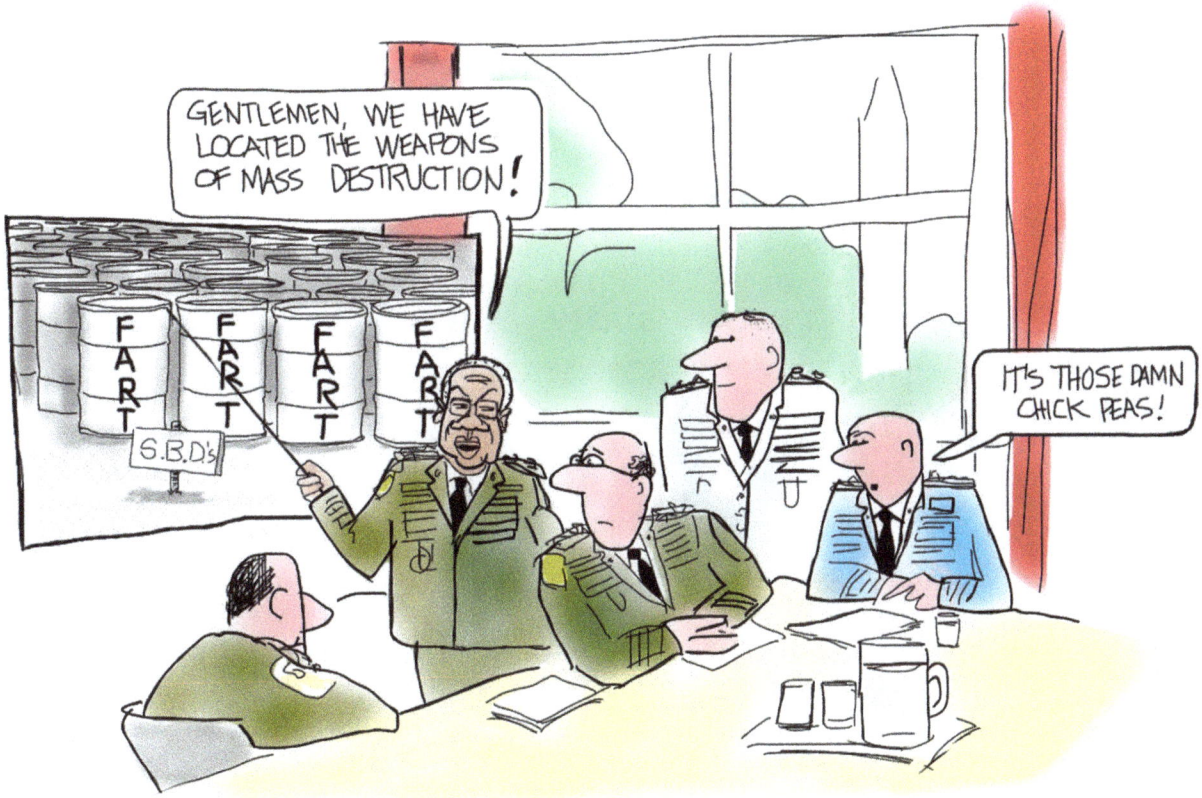

That's a pretty shitty joke
"Butt" don't blame me,
It's my rectum's show
And he thinks it's funny.

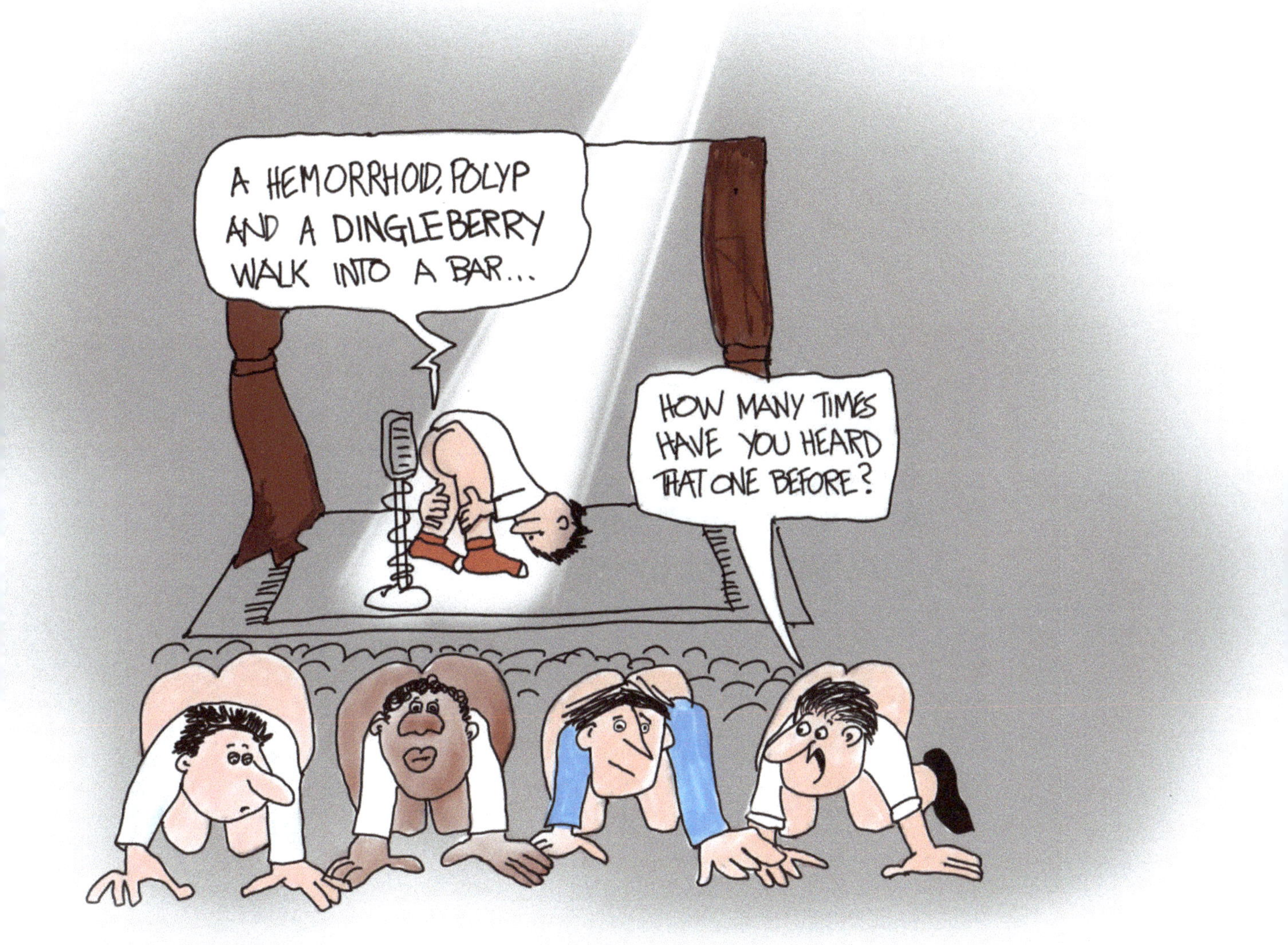
A HEMORRHOID, POLYP AND A DINGLEBERRY WALK INTO A BAR...
HOW MANY TIMES HAVE YOU HEARD THAT ONE BEFORE?

Colonoscopy isn't
A warm, friendly word.
And how humiliating if they found
A 13-year old turd?

A 13 YEAR OLD TURD ??
HOW CAN YOU TELL?
I'M WATCHING ITS
BAR MITZVAH.

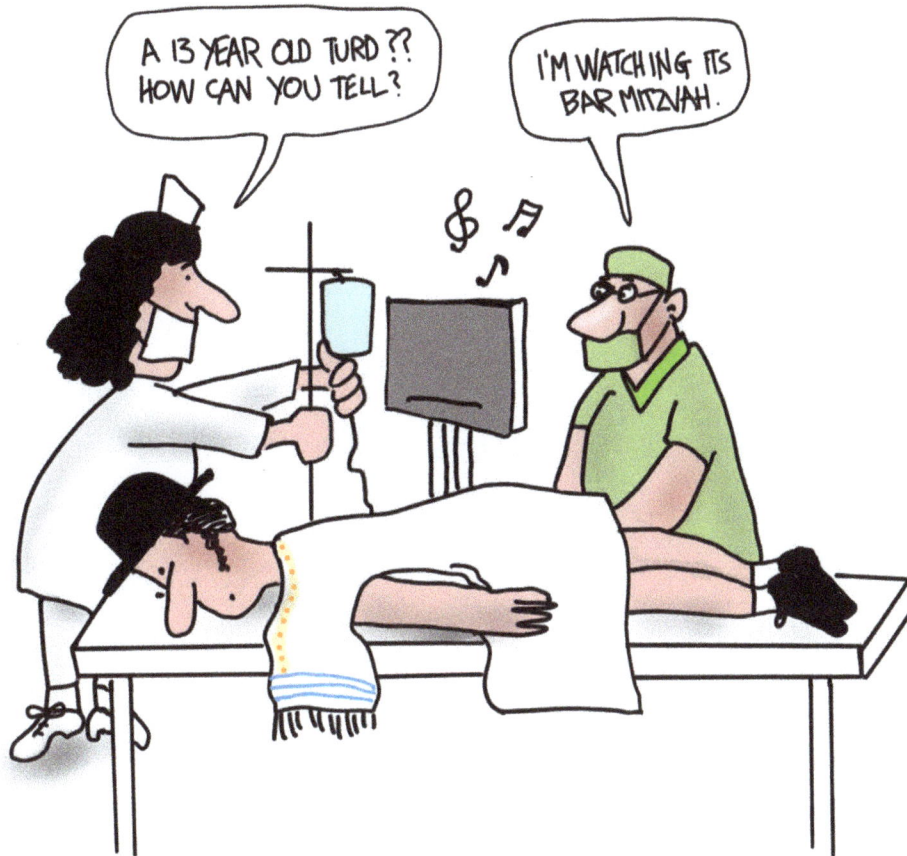

Yes, I wanted to avoid cancer,
And polyps and such,
Yet 6-feet of exploring,
Seemed a bit much.

BIG SMILE AND PLUMP YOURSELF UP. THIS VIDEO WILL BE VIRAL BY MORNING.

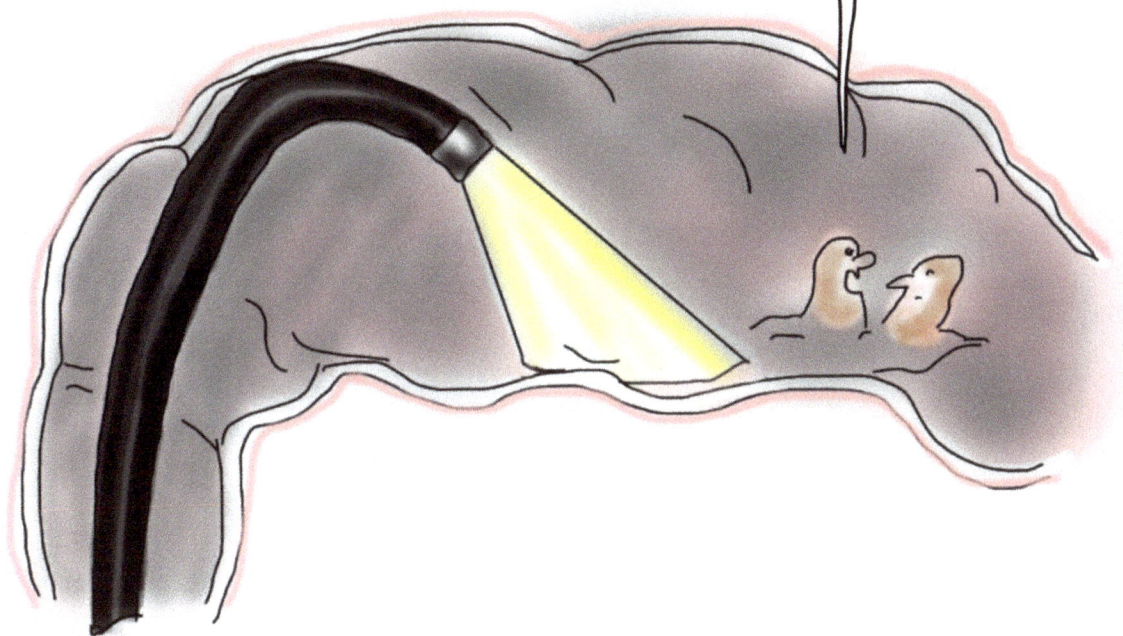

6-feet of hose
Came as quite a shock.
It sent millions more shivers
Right through my (rhymes with sock).

TO MAKE SURE EVERYTHING IS WORKING ON THE COUNT OF THREE, TURN AROUND.

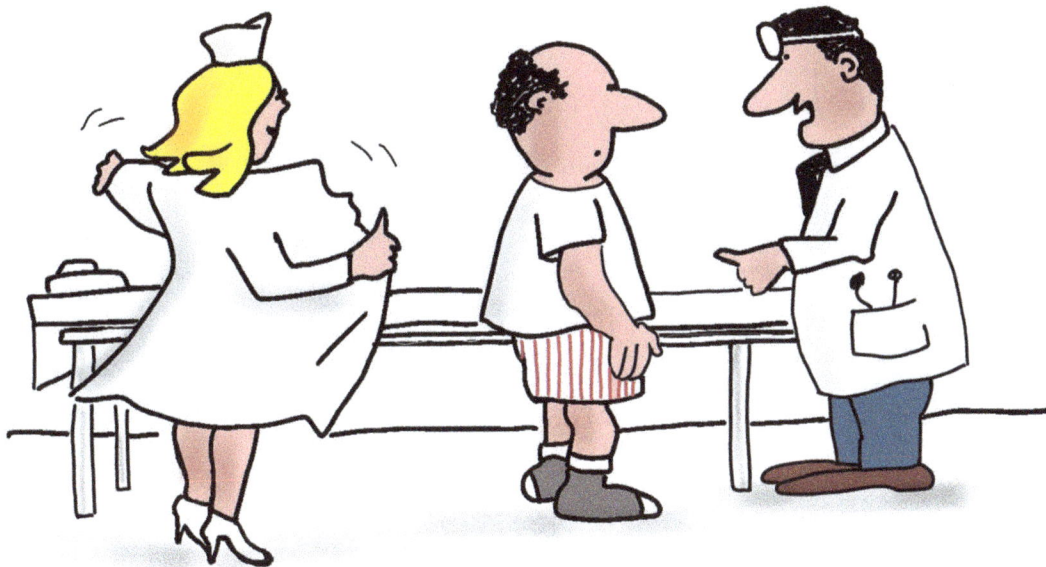

My first colonoscopy
With my ass on TV,
Maybe my a-hole and doctor
Would take a selfie?

CRACK A SMILE.

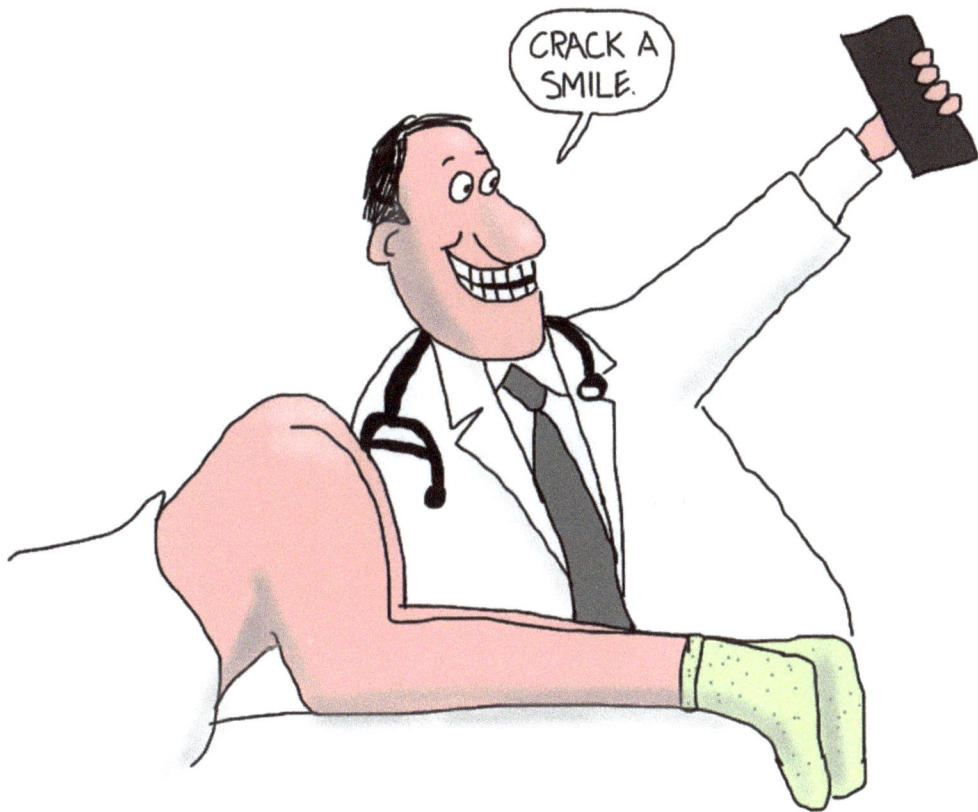

When I awoke from the procedure
The doc stood smiling at me.
I said, "What's with the racing gloves?"
He said, "It was like the friggin' Grand Prix!"

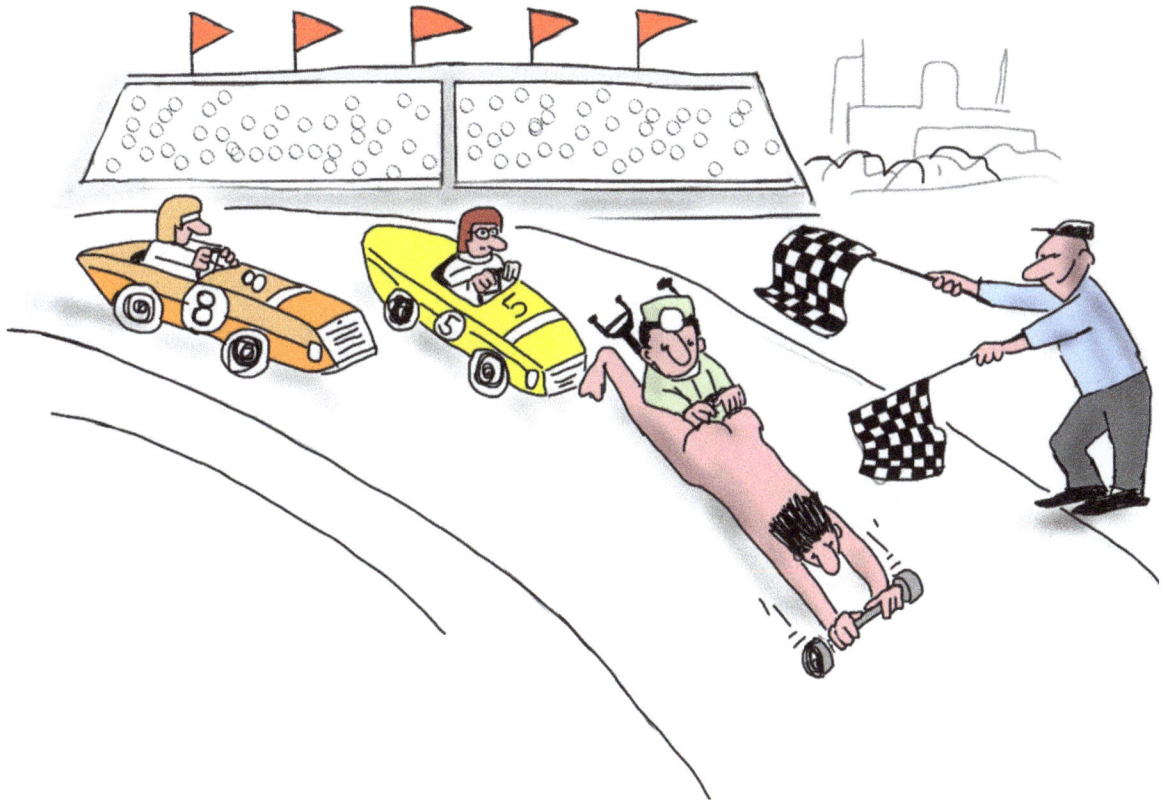

Said he never met an asshole
That was so squeaky clean.
He complimented me profusely
On my anal hygiene.

JACKPOT!!!
COLONOSCOPY ROOM

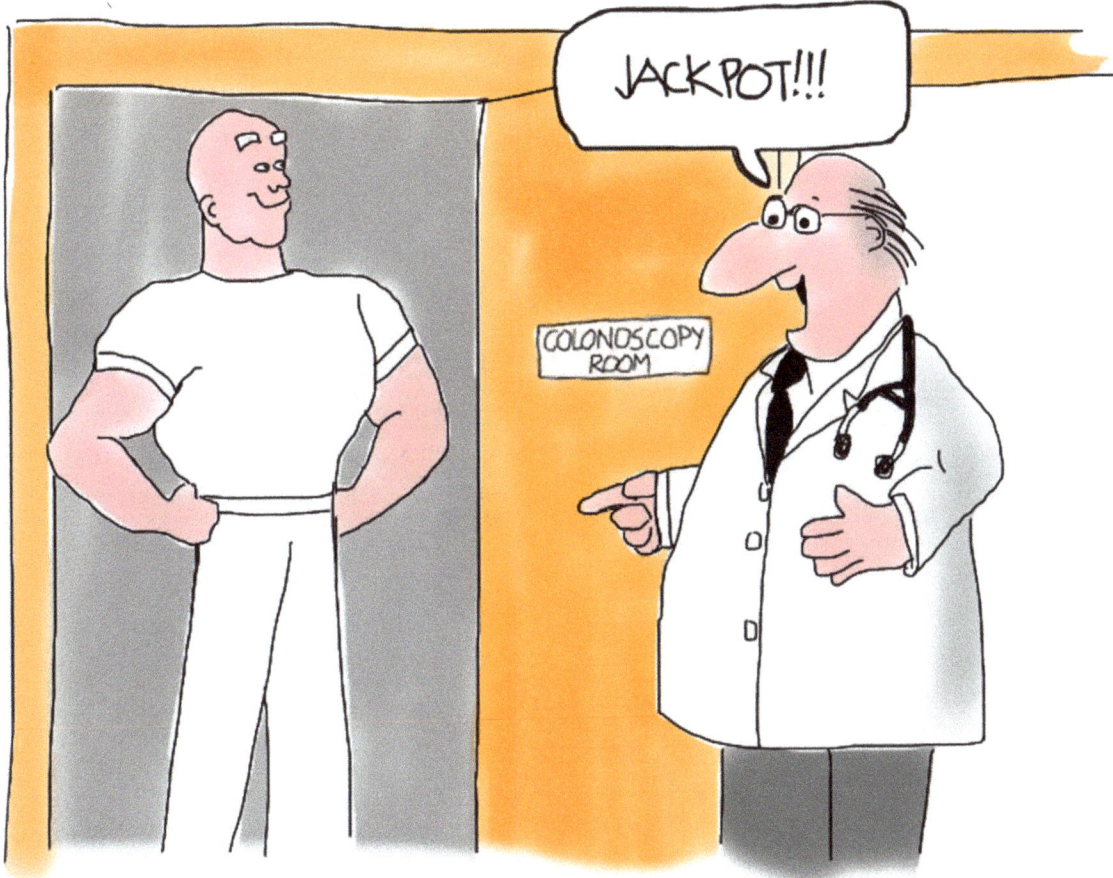

It was time to go celebrate,
Bump fists, hoist some beers.
But first I'll schedule my colonoscopy
With my doc in 10 years.

WOW, IT'S 10 YEARS ALREADY? SEEMS LIKE ONLY 4 CARTOONS AGO.

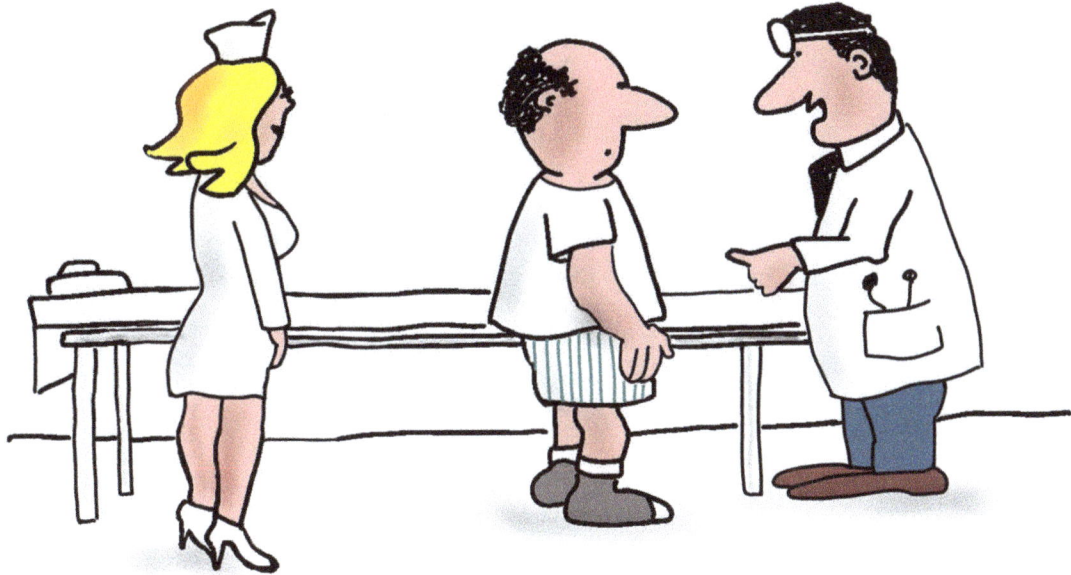

So, my advice to you all
May seem a bit crass,
Should you schedule yours now?
You bet your sweet fuc*#!g ass!

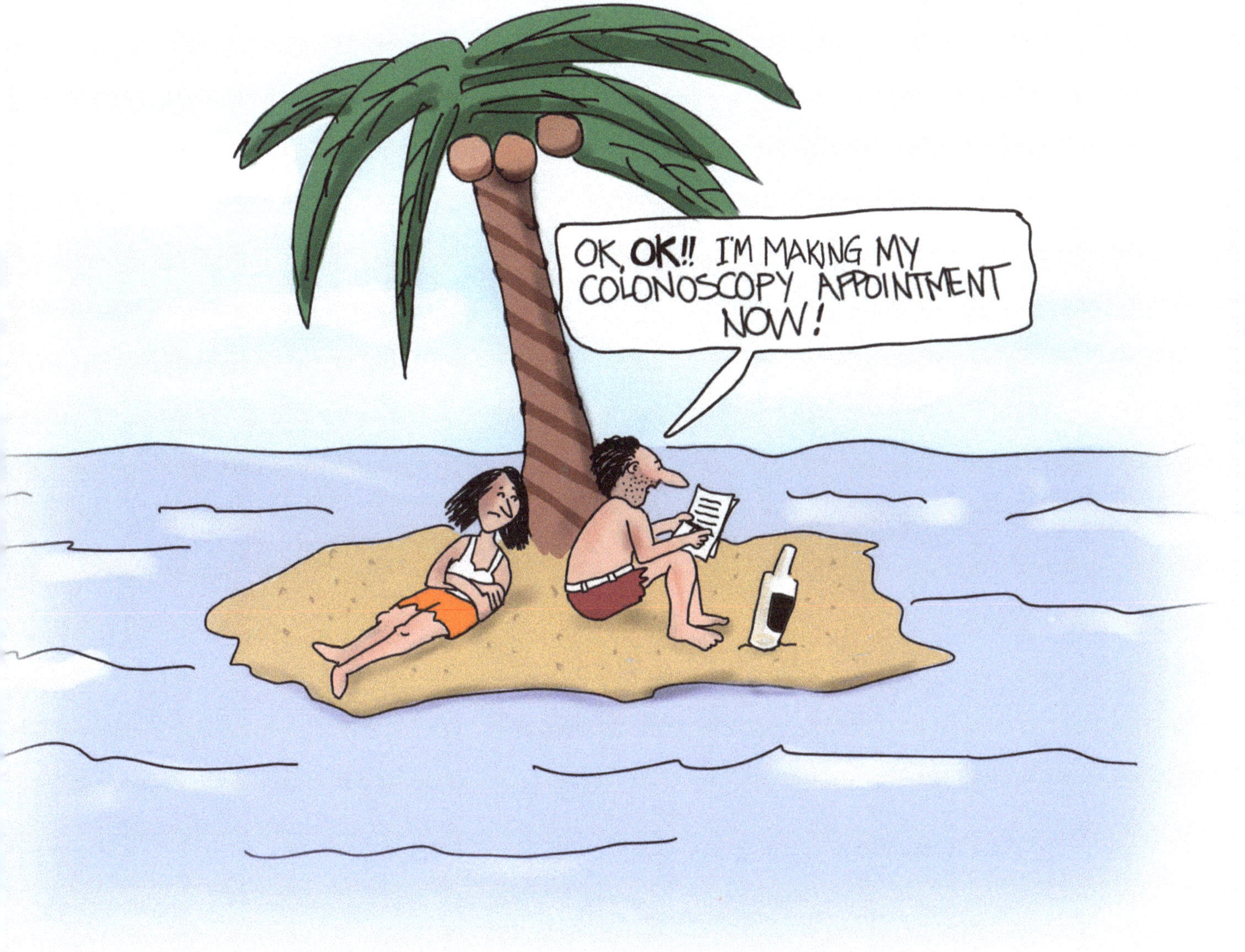
OK, OK!! I'M MAKING MY COLONOSCOPY APPOINTMENT NOW!

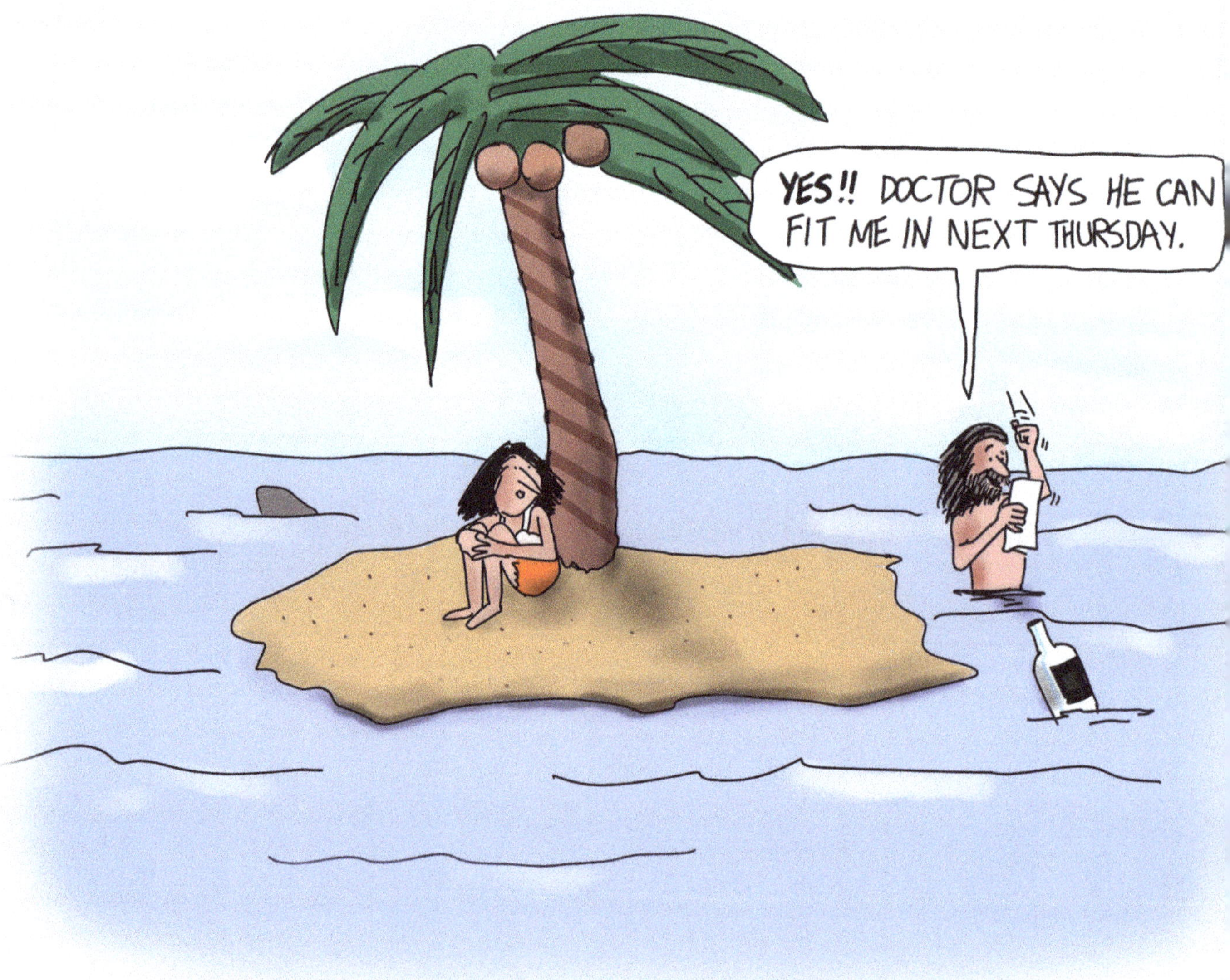
YES!! DOCTOR SAYS HE CAN FIT ME IN NEXT THURSDAY.

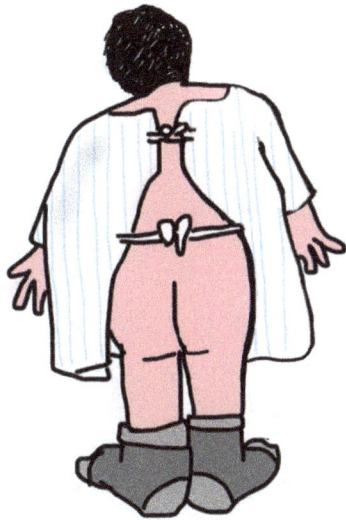

THE END.

ASSDENDUM

Almost 15 million colonoscopies are performed each year. Well, add one to that number because it's your turn! The recommended age of a first colonoscopy used to be 50. A slew of medical evidence proved that getting one at age 45 could save lots more lives. So, 45 is *not* the new 35, it's the new 50.

OMG. Wait, that's you! You've hit 45. Or 50. Or older. Time to go from Jello shots to Jello prep!

If you think those first 45 years flew by in the blink of an eye, you'll soon be the person who has fallen and can't get up. YEP! You. And you know what it's time for if you want to live to a ripe old age?

Your First Colonoscopy!

Yes, you. Don't look left or right. We're talking to you! Or someone who's buying this for you as a present (it makes a wonderful birthday gift).

What you've lost in muscle tissue at your age you've hopefully gained in wisdom. Still not convinced? Don't do it for you!

Do it for your kid's sake.
Do it for your wife or husband's sake.
Do it for your partner's sake.
Do it for your best friend's sake.
Do it for god's sake.

Even better, do it for our sake. Bob* and Mal .**
We'd really like to sell some books!

*Bob has had 3 colonoscopies. The first found 2 polyps that were removed on the spot that could have become cancers. Saved his ass. His second and third were nice and clean. It's time for a 4th. He's getting so used to it, he's having a toilet named after him. The "Bob-A-Loo."

**Mal has had 2 colonoscopies. 2 polyps were found the first time. Whoosh! All gone. And he is very excited about getting his third one in a few years. He really loves Jello.

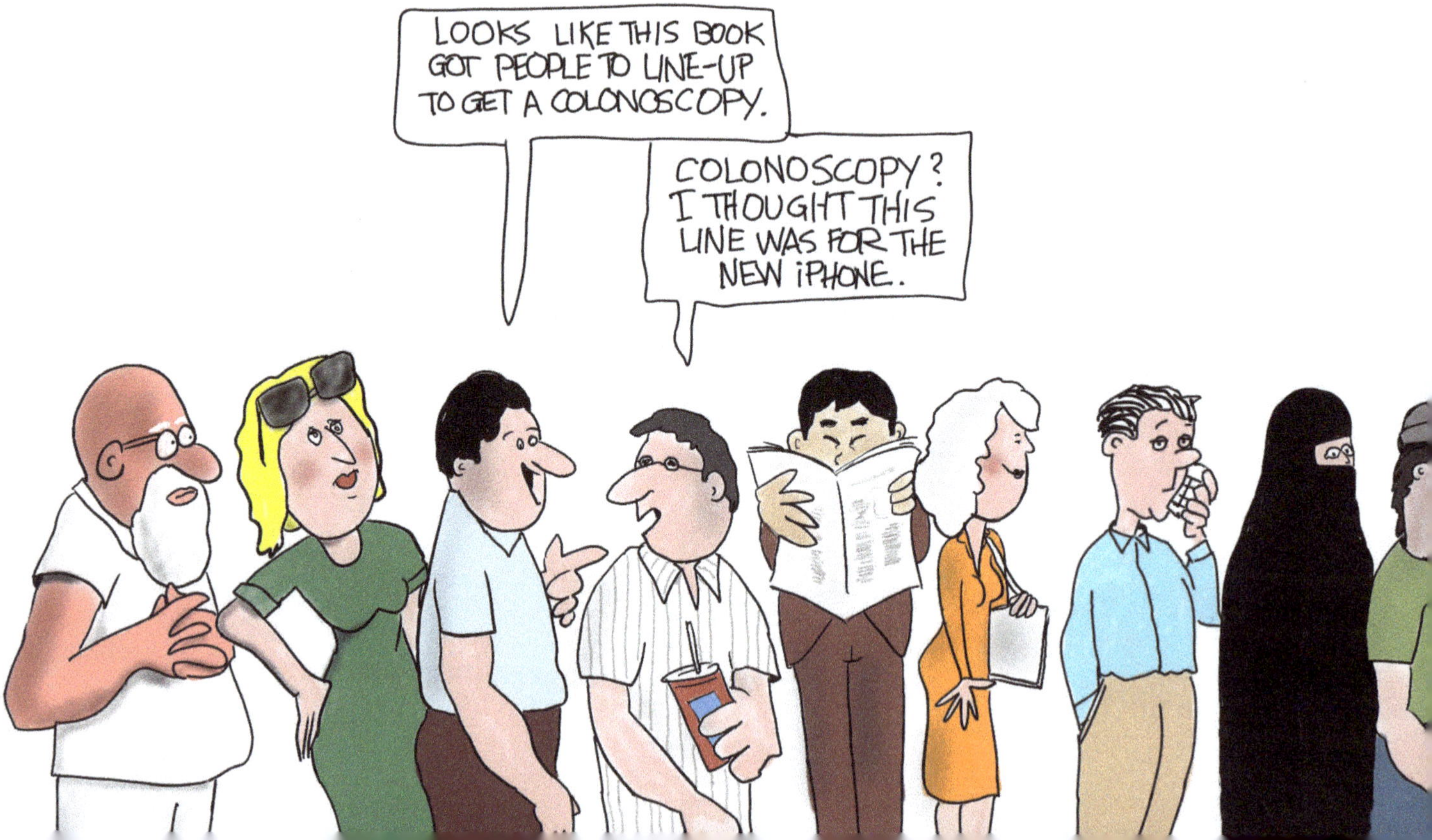
LOOKS LIKE THIS BOOK GOT PEOPLE TO LINE-UP TO GET A COLONOSCOPY.
COLONOSCOPY? I THOUGHT THIS LINE WAS FOR THE NEW iPHONE.

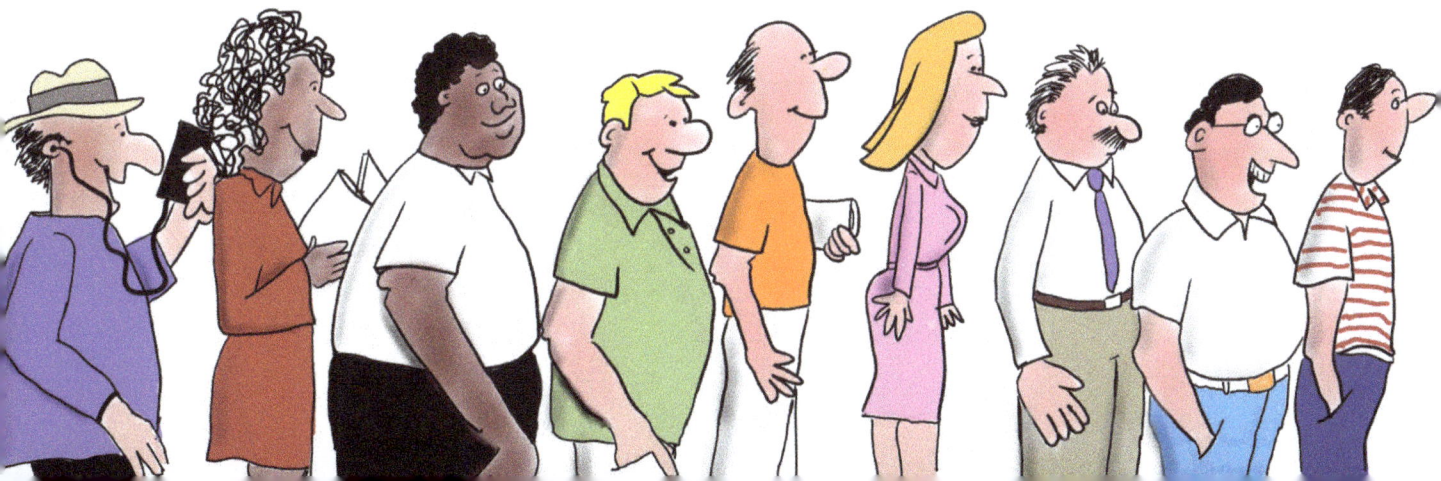

www.ingramcontent.com/pod-product-compliance
Lightning Source LLC
Chambersburg PA
CBHW040245100426

42811CB00011B/1162